I0115731

MEDICAL MISADVENTURE 2

STOLEN IDENTITY

..THE PROBLEM WITH THE LAW…

BY SEMISI PONE
BSc, MSc (Hons)

Copyright © Rainbow Enterprises Books

Publisher: Rainbow Enterprises Books

ISBN:978-1-98-851112-2

All rights reserved. No part of this book shall be
reproduced, in any way, without prior written
permission from the writer and copyright holder.

INTRODUCTION

This book complements the first book
MEDICAL MISADVENTURE, a sufferer's
account, it is also about a huge legal problem
which caused so much trouble for me that it still
not resolved today, after 20 years. I feel it is not
really my fault and I hope this book will shed
some light on it.

I wanted to discuss 1. first my problem with a
vaccine injury in 1996 (already published in
MEDICAL MISADVENTURE, a sufferer's
account (available from amazon.com) which is
still affecting my health today 2. I also want to
discuss some legal issues which still affect me
to-day as book 2 of this same Medical
Misadventure Issue. No one knows about these
problems apart from a few professional people
and close family.

Why would I want to discuss such a very
sensitive issue? It is because I feel that the best
way to deal with these 'underlying problems' is
to expose them for what they are.

I would like to apologize to the people named in
this book, if they are offended , in any way, but I
have to record these events as truthfully as
possible.

CHAPTER 1. The Beginning

After I had decided to stay in Auckland, I informed the South Pacific Commission (SPC) Secretary General, Bob Dunne (Australia) that I will not be coming back to my job in Fiji.

I rang him first in April 1996. I wanted to know whether there has been a decision made regarding my job as Plant Protection Advisor and Co-ordinator of the SPC Plant Protection Service. Bob said that he does not know what is happening. He has just joined SPC a few months before but he will look into it. He will check with the Human Resources people whether they have selected a candidate. All the SPC 'core budget' staff positions had been advertised a year earlier but there has been no decision made, in my case.

> I was told 'advertising our jobs' was a 'restructuring exercise', which smacks of 'stupidity' in my view. Why would you advertise all the jobs and rehire them again? It seems to be such a waste of time.

Bob knows me already from our meeting in Suva when he came around to meet the staff , on his appointment a few months earlier, and we made presentations on our projects. It has been many months since we applied for our jobs with no decisions made.

Further to this problem of job insecurity was my health problem after the vaccination. I had no idea whether I will still have a job and whether my dizziness will go away. It was beginning to scare me. Anyone, blacking out regular would be scared. Even if they give me my job back, I might have some major issues with my health in Fiji.

I decided to fax Bob a short note to say, I am withdrawing my application and I will not be coming back. I will stay in Auckland. I did not tell him about my health problem because I did not know what it is…and the Doctor already told me that I am fine.

I have discussed most of that in the first book. MEDICAL MISADVENTURE, a sufferer's account.

Starting a business

After unsuccessfully looking for a job, I decided to start a business. I registered a company and began trading in Auckland.

My business failed in the first year. I have been reading a lot before going into business that 95% of small businesses in New Zealand will fail in the first 2 years, but I was confident of succeeding. The first few months made me realize that there is something else going on.

The shop that I bought was not making any money from its main business of fruits and vegetables, with a small amount of groceries. My plan was to introduce some root crops, and other produce, from the Pacific Islands which will help Pacific growers market their produce, and turn the shop profitability around. In fact, my sales doubled in the first few months after my first container of cassava arrived from Fiji.

I also looked around for other opportunities.

I made some enquiries and discovered from my lawyer, Mr Sione Fonua, that an old rugby mate, Savelio Fonoimoana, from Eden Rugby Football Club, Sandringham, Auckland is looking for investors. He was doing well manufacturing and selling coconut cream from a factory at Henderson Valley. I went to see his factory and I took some of his coconut cream products home to try. They were very good. I was convinced we will make a good profit out of it. He told me he is importing his coconuts from Tuvalu in 20 kg sacks but they are irregular and sometimes spoilage can be a problem. That was the limiting factor for his business.

> I was looking at both options at the same time. That is, the shop and coconut cream production and decided to invest in both.

I offered to supply him with all the coconuts he will need. He accepted my offer. It was all done with a handshake like old rugby mates.

I flew to Tonga to organize the coconuts. I discussed it with my family and they agreed to do it. I will pay them ten cents for each nut plus shipping and extra costs. I also bought a $6,000 3 tonne truck for them to use in Tonga. It was all organized and I flew back to Auckland.

In exactly one month, the first container with 30,000 coconuts arrived. That was about August, 1996. Another container with 30,000 nuts arrived in September 1996. I had invoiced Mr Fonoimoana for $8,000 for the first container then another $8,0000 for the second container. I was charging him about 30 cents per nut. He promised to pay $500 per week.

Another former acquaintance, Mr Talanoa Hala'api'api, also ordered a container of cassava from me. His family are known to us going back a few years. It was done over the phone, like family.

He normally buy his cassava, for supply to customers in Auckland, from Tonga. But he said, that there were no cassava to be found. Tonga cannot supply him with any cassava. His business was going down. I ordered a container of cassava for him from my supplier in Fiji.

Problems began in about October-November when both my business partners (Mr Fonoimoana and Mr Hala'api'api) cannot pay me. I was not relying on the shop sales because I knew before I started that I will have to make money from other sales…and not shop sales, even though shop sales reached more than $600 plus in one day equating to about $4,000 in sales a week. The turnover when I took over was less than $1,000 a week

I sought advice from many people and the conclusion was, I should take Mr Fonoimoana to court over the $16,000 unpaid bill. He has promised to pay many times but nothing eventuated.

I talked to many lawyers and they recommended Mr John Long, a lawyer in the CBD. I was asked to make a deposit of $1700 before proceedings started. I paid the money to a lawyer Roger O'Donell at Sunnynook and provided all the

paper work, including signed statements by Mr
Fonoimoana that he will pay the full amount.
However, I was still required to go through a
'discovery process' where another female lawyer
took notes on what happened. The time it took
and other processes blew the budget to more
than $3,000. Mr Fonoimoana also wrote to me
and requested whether we should cancel the
court case because he has also run out of funds
to pay for his lawyers. I agreed.

> The Disputes Tribunal at the time only allow for
> claims of up to $3,000.

Mr Fonoimoana had used one container (30,000
coconuts) and sold the cream, so why has he not
paid?

I decided to dig a bit deeper and found that he
owes a lot of money to the Pacific Business
Facility (an organization helping Pacific
Islanders to start businesses) which lend him the
cash to start his business. Was he selling the
cream from 30,000 coconuts to pay his debt?
I also found out that Mr Fonoimoana had 2
properties under his name which raises the
question as to why he refused to pay.

> At the time I was aware of a rumor there is a woman using
> my name who used to live in Otara but later moved to
> Henderson. Was she behind it?

Mr Hala'api'api also could not pay the $6,000
for the container of frozen Fijian cassava. He
decided to return the container of cassava after
2-3 weeks. He said that it was 'woody', which is
a problem with some cassava roots that weren't
processed properly. The cassava roots normally
have a 'woody' part where it is attached to the
cassava stem. This part has to be cut off during
processing, but sometimes process workers do
not cut them off completely and it does reduce
the quality of the frozen root for consumption. I
checked the cassava from that container and
although there was 5% of it that was woody, it
was otherwise alright. I arranged with a Fijian
customer, Sam Lotawa, who was buying cassava
regularly to sell the container for me.

I authorized the Freezer Warehouse Manager to
deal directly with Sam who will buy the frozen
bags of cassava off him and sell them. It worked
very well. Sam sold all the cassava in the
warehouse!.

Mr Hala'api'api also moved his operation to the
Henderson valley from his Grey Lynn house. He set up
shop just about 50 metres from Mr Fonoimoana's factory.
Suspicious? I think so.

By January 1997, I had exhausted my cash
supply and the shop sales of $2-4,000 a week did

not generate enough profits to pay for everything.

The court case could not persuade Mr Fonoimoana to pay and Mr Hala'api'api was not very helpful either. I decided to close down the business. My health had deteriorated to the point where I was completely exhausted by the time I closed the shop at 6pm. The dizziness did not help. Blacking out momentarily, in the shop, several times a day was not very conducive to business success.

I sold the shop for $750 after buying it for $16,000 and canceled my lease. I was not in a position, physically and mentally, to sit in the shop and wait for some Good Samaritan to buy it at a premium price. There were some good selling points, like the new root crop products and new delivery customers, but the landlord had also advised that the rent will increase from $16,000 to $24,000 in the following year. That killed the chicken before the egg was laid.

Mr Fonoimoana's landlord called me and asked me to remove the 20,000 plus coconuts sitting in his factory. He is kicking Mr Fonoimoana out of there for not paying his rent. I told him that I had sold them to Mr Fonoimoana. He is the owner of those coconuts. Mr Fonoimoana owes me $16,000 for the 60,000 coconuts supplied and he has not paid.

I had tried many times to help Mr Fonoimoana save his business. I offered to provide a young man to do all the processing work for him, but after organizing everything he did not turn up in the morning to pickup his worker! Twice!

Health supplements

I had started taking supplements like aloe vera juice, anti-oxidant tablets and fish oil. That is probably what saved me. I saw this very short advert in the NZ Herald, 'Be Healthy and Wealthy' with a phone number. I called and she came with some of her products to 'show and tell' what it was all about. It was my introduction to Network Marketing which was taking New Zealand by storm. Carol Stephenson, was a nice lady, who used to do real estate but now sell health products. I did try my hand at Network Marketing for a while.

The coconut cream factory closed down

Somebody called me a few weeks after I closed my shop whether I want Mr Fonoimoana's equipment. I told them I don't because he should sell them and pay me the money. I never heard back from them. The landlord probably sold them to recover rental arrears.

Some years later when the Indonesian coconut cream Kara hit the New Zealand market, it did occur to a few people how much money we could have made from Mr Fonoimoana's concentrated coconut cream, but it was too late.

Reviving a poorly operated business

Mr Hala'api'api also called and asked whether I can give him some cassava from Fiji, again. There was just no cassava from Tonga. I had considered his business. He was buying his cassava, and probably yams, from relatives in Tonga. The Chief of their village is my second cousin. I am related, through ancestry, to many of the people from that village. I thought that I should help him to succeed, because it would give my relatives a market for their root crops in New Zealand. I gave him two names of suppliers I was dealing with in Fiji. A very successful businessman named Michael Joe and my friend John Sanday who had supplied the first container of frozen Fijian cassava to Mr Hala'api'api.

I heard Mr Hala'api'api is still in business today (2018) after 20 years from that conversation….and I am happy to say he is still importing root crops from the village.

I was not in a position to carry on with the business because of my health problems.

Buyers of the shop

There were a couple of Chinese immigrants who came to New Zealand about the same time as us. They wanted to buy our shop, but I had advised them not to. The new rent of $24,000 a year is just too much.

I further advised them to sell vegetables at the fairs and gave them the truck in exchange for their car. They bought their veges from Turners and Growers. After a few weeks, they said they were making $800 per day at the fair after just a few weeks of trading! That was much more than what I was making in one day!

Some good was coming out of my disaster!

CHAPTER 2. The woman in my shoes

The rumor of the woman just won't go away. Now they tell me that she has $999 million in her bank account. What was worse, my father also confirmed the rumors.

The rumors

I analyzed the story and concluded the following;

1. The woman is using my name
2. She has $999 million in the bank
3. The money was possibly a lottery I won in the USA for $US365# million (the exchange rate was about $US1 to $NZ3)
4. They have set up the account so I can have easy access and 'safe cover' from other people who might 'cheat me'.

I went to the bank and sure enough I have an account under my name there. I was given a bank card, but the bank clerk said the money had been removed and taken to Tonga!

- I spent a night in Los Angeles on my way to London in 1995 and I bought a lottery ticket there in the hotel reception for $US20. My wallet, including the lottery ticket, was stolen some weeks later at the Mocambo Hotel, Nadi, Fiji.

The Addresses

The address on the bank account was 39 Cobham Crescent, Otara. The title on the account was a Ms.

I drove to the address and sat on the opposite side of the road and watched the house for about an hour. A Pacific Island woman came outside but I did not recognize her.

I also drove to another address, which I found in the phone book, at 36 Larissa Place, Henderson and watched the house for an hour but there was no one there, at the time.

Again I was told that the account is locked and I have to open it....and so I deposited some money into the account and waited, but nothing happened after 2 weeks. I thought the woman using my name would use the money.

I withdrew the money and deposited more money and went to visit my parents in Tonga. I have not seen them for several years. I would also ask around, if anyone knows anything about the $999 million.

I also opened an account in Auckland, before I left, with another bank, and put some money there. My idea was that whoever is using my name will probably come after me. She will raid my accounts and maybe try other 'punishments'.

The Tongan Health Episode

In Tonga, I did not find anyone with information about the $999 million. During that trip I was driving home one day in my Dad's ute and I completely lost feeling in my arms and legs about a kilometre from home. I was able to move them, and get the ute home, but I cannot feel anything! I had to return to Auckland because of that health scare.

The Police

In Auckland, I had the biggest shock of my life when the Police turned up, early one morning, and arrested me for using that account with the 39 Cobham Crescent, Otara address. It seems that the account holder was a Police Officer! What was he doing using my name and a woman's title? And why did they send the $999 million to Tonga? …and where was the money from? Was it true that they stole my lotto money?

The Nuthouse

To make a long story short, the judge found that I may be 'nuts' and should be put in the crazy house for observation. So they put me in the nuthouse for a few weeks to check whether I have gone completely off the rail. After two weeks they let me go home, I think they changed their minds, I am not really crazy. I was put in one of the community service programmes for the disabled for a few years for 'rehabilitation'.

I suspect that they found some 'bugs' in my blood and had to 'treat me' for 2 weeks. After those 2 weeks in the nuthouse I felt much better. Whatever caused me to lose feelings in my arms and legs for almost 2 hours, in Tonga, was completely gone.

I was also told that it was some 'other patient' and it was not me. I was getting a bit confused.

The $10 million

Upon returning home from the hospital, I had another shock. The Police had taken all my bank cheque books and bank cards before the court case but I found a bank statement in the rubbish at home. The new bank account I opened before leaving to Tonga had $10 million in it. The problem was, the Police has all the bank cards

and cheque books! Who was the beneficiary?
Who ended up with the $999 million and the $10
million? Only the New Zealand Police can tell
us.

Long term health problems

My health has not improved at all after 20 years.
It has deteriorated, probably with age, as well as
gout and arthritic symptoms. They are consistent
with vaccine injury symptoms as explained in
the first book MEDICAL MISADVENTURE, a
sufferer's account.

The problem now is that they have added mental
health to my repertoire of illnesses. Once people
think you may be nuts, there is an uphill battle
for the rest of your life.

Rubbish Claims

I know many people will rubbish my claims.
That they are all 'made up'. That is why I
include the names of many people in this book
so they can confirm my stories.

CHAPTER 3. My Assessment of the Problems

When my health problems got a bit worse, I was told to just 'harden up'. I thought it was a joke. But it is probably the only thing one can do is to 'harden up' and not let the health problems interfere with living a normal life.

Questions

The question is why did all these 'things' happen. It was obvious that somebody was in the background 'pulling the strings'. I don't let it bother me much, but there is some kind of insistence in it…that I should be controlled by 'them'. I am not paranoid but it does fuel the mental health fire.

I am writing this story because it needs to be written. We have to look at the issues raised and ask the right questions. What is it all about? Was it some kind of punishment by a greater power? What did I do to offend those people?

Obviously, it had something to do with my job as Plant Protection Advisor, and Co-ordinator of the Plant Protection Service, at the South Pacific Commission. I am not sure what it was, but somebody did get angry enough to sabotage my job and my business. Hopefully, they did not interfere with the vaccine or it will raise some really 'ugly' questions. For example, did somebody interfere with the vaccine that killed two babies in Samoa just last month?.

I have already mentioned in the first book that I decided to tell this story because of the two babies that died of vaccine injuries in Samoa. We have to talk about the problems in the Pacific region and raise awareness to protect children and adults alike, from future injuries by vaccination.

The South Pacific Commission (SPC is now known as the Secretariat for the Pacific Community) is a huge organization with 27 member countries. The list of countries is included in the first book MEDICAL MISADVENTURE, a sufferer's account. The SPC has a large Health Programme which work with all 22 Pacific Island members on health issues. They will be the right people to lead such a campaign. That is, to make vaccination safer.

Was it envy?

There has been many comments that insinuated that I was the 'wrong person' for the job, by other Pacific Islanders, during my time at SPC.

However, if you read all my publications on PLANT PROTECTION IN THE PACIFIC books 1-4 (all available from amazon.com), you will realize immediately, that I have more experience in the Pacific Islands…than any other candidate…in the field of Plant Protection. I still have a few more books to write on the work I did during 10 years in Plant Protection in Tonga, Samoa and Fiji. No other Pacific Island candidate has that amount of Plant Protection work done, in the Pacific Islands, at senior level before 1993, when I took over as Plant Protection Advisor at the South Pacific Commission.

It was obvious, I was the right candidate.

Was it alcohol?

I have been told also that I consume too much alcohol while at the South Pacific Commission. However, I like to point out….the only time I consume alcohol was after work and during the weekends. It is well known that Pacific Islanders tend to be a bit noisy after a few beers. It happens everywhere, including Auckland, but I don't think we should assess our staff on their 'after hours' performance.

Was it Kava?

At the South Pacific Commission, Suva Campus, as everywhere in Fiji, during 1993-1996, staff are allowed to drink kava during work hours. It is a Fijian tradition and no one criticize kava drinking during work hours.

I prefer not to drink kava during work hours except on the occasion that I visit a MAFF or other office and they offer me a kava bowl which I will accept because it is a tradition with them. They offer their visitors a kava shell before they talk.

Was it incompetence?

I was co-ordinating more than 30 million dollars worth of projects and I personally managed a $5 million project. A list is in the first book MEDICAL MISADVENTURE, a sufferer's account (amazon.com). All these projects were renewed or approved during my time at SPC.

I also managed to get the Pacific Plant Protection Organization (PPPO) established after 8 years of discussion among member countries.

The list of things that I was able to do during 3 years, at SPC, is mind boggling. It also amazed me as well.

Only Superman could have done better.

Was it disagreements with other staff?

All professional staff , in large organizations,
around the world disagree on many things. It is a
healthy way to operate. What the management
should do is find ways for 'staff dispute' to be
sorted.

I always stand up for my department and I don't
like to compromise our projects in favor of
cutting workloads or resolutions for future
operations. One such dispute had to be resolved
by the Director of Services, Mrs Fusi
Taginavanua. I disagreed with the Manager of
the Agriculture Programme, Dr Malcolm
Hazelman, on budget allocations. As the
Co-ordinator of the Plant Protection Service, I
feel it is my job and my budget. There is a very
clear responsibility role regarding the budgets. I
am the one responsible, but when I want to
spend the money, management has to approve it
first.

I don't see any problem disagreeing with
Managers or other staff. I mean, I cannot agree
to everything they propose…because I already
have project documents that dictate how and
where the money should be spent. For example,
my SPC/EU $5 million project, I have to report
to the European Union Office in Suva, every

quarter, how we are spending the money! I cannot tell them that other staff at SPC are spending the money for me! I have to strictly follow the project document that was approved by the SPC, EU and Forum Secretariat.

Some of our projects were given to other organizations. I would not have agreed to it.

For example, when I left SPC, our biggest project was a $NZ 24 million project on biodiversity/systematics, in collaboration with Professor Tecwyn Jones of the Commonwealth Agriculture Bureau (CAB International, UK), was handed over to the University of the South Pacific. The SPC and CAB International funded the $US200,000 regional meetings to discuss the project and put together the proposal for funding, but somebody decided 'on his own' to give the project to the USP when the funds were approved. That was after I had left SPC.

I would not have done that if I was still the Co-ordinator. What I would do is give some of the systematics work to the USP to do…and provide the funds. But I will keep control of the project (It was called PACINET or Pacific Biosystematics Network).

It is clear from this short discussion that many disagreements can occur, at SPC, when other staff try to spent your project money....because you are the person responsible!

The Food and Agriculture Organization (FAO) of the United Nations

I would like to mention my work with the FAO because I was due to attend a meeting of the experts on Biosecurity (Phytosanitary Measures) in May 1996. I was unable to go because I felt that my health problem may interfere with such a long flight from Auckland to Rome, where the meeting was at FAO HQ.

I faxed Dr Niek van der Graff, the FAO Chief of Plant Protection and organizer of our meeting, and told him I cannot come. I did not tell him about my health scare because as mentioned already, I was not really sure what it was that caused the 'momentary black outs'.

Was it just fate? Some bad karma?

I think that it could have been some bad luck...but also helped along by some 'opportunists'.

I don't dwell on it but the story need to be told.

I think that everyone should get their facts right. Everything I have written in books 1 & 2 of MEDICAL MISADVENTURE is true. There would be no point of writing anything if it was all lies.

I should mention my suspicions here, as well.

There is a possibility that the $999 million was a joke or hoax. Why?

It seems to be a 'numbers' game.

For example, the number 365 is the number of the Police Station at Glenfield, Auckland.

The number of the Police woman who arrested me is 391. The number 999 is an analogy of 39....that is there are 3x9s!

Whoever spends time thinking up an elaborate joke like that must be very, very clever in a lunatic way!

The $10 million cannot be a hoax, it was on my Bank Statement unless the Bank Statement was just 'made up' on somebody's computer....and then conveniently dropped at our house for me to find.

Finally, I have deliberately left out the names of Police Officers and some other information which does not add anything to this story....but might inflame the situation further. That is not the objective of the books. The objective is to highlight the problem of vaccine injury.

www.ingramcontent.com/pod-product-compliance
Lightning Source LLC
Chambersburg PA
CBHW021340290326
41933CB00038B/996